Grain Belly, Wheat Brain

HEATH EASTON

ISBN: 1507731132
ISBN-13: 978-1507731130

TWO THANK YOU GIFTS

As a Thank You to readers for buying this book we put together two free gifts to help you on your *Grain Belly, Wheat Brain* journey

These gifts were created for you to print off and keep handy in the kitchen, so visit the link below to get access.

www.BlueBeanpublishing.com/Gluten-Free

TABLE OF CONTENTS

INTRODUCTION

Despite all of our achievements in the developed world, public health is still as big a problem as ever. The obesity epidemic continues unabated and related health issues like diabetes, heart disease and cancer are pushing healthcare systems and national budgets to the breaking point.

It is a particularly disturbing problem for the average Joe. Despite an explosion in the popularity of personal fitness, health, nutrition and exercise, public health trends for the future paint a worrying picture.

Half of American adults are expected to be obese by 2030 (compared to only 15% in 1960)[1,2], . Worldwide, deaths from diabetes are projected to double between

2005 and 2030[3]. In spite of our advanced understanding of biology and nutrition and a greater interest in personal health and fitness by individuals and national organizations, the outlook for the health of the average American or European is bleak.

So what are we missing? Why are things getting worse, despite our best efforts?

The answer may surprise you.

Gluten, and more specifically wheat, represents the most profound and insidious threat to public health in the developed world. Recent findings by doctors and scientists are pointing to the fact that despite the privileged position wheat and gluten products enjoy in our diets, there isn't a single cell in the human body that escapes their negative effects.

The consumption of gluten and wheat has been associated with a whole host of conditions affecting every organ in your body. From the obvious connection to conditions that were thought to have no relation to diet whatsoever – until recently.

What's most scary for the average family is the way that wheat has undergone drastic biochemical changes over the last 60 years, without any form of safety testing. This new age wheat has become part of our daily lives - few foods have reached the level of ubiquity in western diets to rival that of wheat. Omnipresent across the world, in all cuisines and cultures, wheat is consumed everywhere and in all shapes and sizes.

It's scary, but at the same time inspiring – this dangerous food that is such a health threat is woven into the fabric of our daily lives, but this also means cutting it out can yield massive benefits.

So, let's dig in and take a look at how we can start taking back our health. We'll take a look at what's inside wheat and learn how wheat has gone through unprecedented changes over the last 50 years. We'll take a tour of the emerging research that shows wheat and gluten as a major culprit in an array of health conditions (and not just celiacs) so you gain awareness of the ways in which your health may be eroding. Most importantly, we'll discuss the best ways to use this knowledge to start improving your health today, with an action plan and some of my favorite recipes.

What's Inside Wheat?

The primary protein found in grains is gluten, which is the ingredient responsible for their shape shifting properties and is the agent that allows bread to rise with yeast and create air pockets for an airy and soft slice of bread. Gluten can be problematic to the digestive system and have certain effects in the rest of the body – It's now fairly well known for its role in celiac disease and gluten sensitivity.

It's important to note that gluten exists in all grains, but that wheat is singled out because it's by far the most prevalent grain our diets, dwarfing consumption of other grains like spelt and barley. Many grains contain problematic gluten, but wheat is the most commonly consumed and also has some uniquely bad characteristics:

For one, there's wheat's affect on blood sugar. While wheat is low fat and contains large amounts of complex carbohydrates and proteins, not all fats, carbohydrates and proteins are the same and similar to milk, has lactose as its primary carbohydrate and casein as its protein. Wheat's main carbohydrate is amylopectin and main protein is gluten.

Amylopectin is indeed a 'complex carbohydrate', which is praised as part of a healthy diet because they tend to be harder to break down and thus, digest slowly, leading to less of a blood sugar spike. Amylopectin is found in different varieties of foods from beans to bananas and also in wheat. They are classified by the rate at which the varieties break down, with amylopectin C (found in beans), digesting slowly and amylopectin B (found in potatoes), digesting at an average complex carbohydrate rate.

The type found in wheat, amylopectin A, is the fastest absorbed variety, and the unique structure of type A allows it to be largely broken down soon after it hits the stomach leading to a quicker and greater impact on blood sugar.

The glycemic index scale, which measures the blood sugar impact from 0-100, with 100 meaning pure glucose and 0 meaning no measurable blood sugar impact, can show the impacts of different carbohydrates. While orange juice and ice cream and potato chips are in the 50s, white bread gets into the 70s, even higher than sucrose (table sugar), which has a GI of 68[4].

This equates to wheat products causing high blood sugar spikes, which as we'll see, have many negative effects on the body. A couple of slices of bread containing about 50 grams of "healthy" complex carbohydrates have essentially the same impact on blood sugar as drinking a regular soda or eating a snickers bar.

A major side effect of the blood sugar high is reduced fullness causing you to be hungry again, much sooner. Also, the dreaded sugar crash is all but unavoidable when eating wheat as the small amount of longer lasting carbohydrate types cannot compensate for the drastic blood sugar plunge once the amylopectin is absorbed by the cells or converted to fat. Low blood sugar following a sugar crash will make you sluggish, irritable and even lightheaded, disoriented and confused.

Wheat's spiking affect on blood sugar (and therefore insulin) along with its problematic proteins like gluten are two of the main ways in which it can wreak havoc on the body. While whole grain wheat has been praised as a healthy part of the diet, forming the base of the nutritional pyramid, the truth is that it's a damaging junk food masquerading as a health food.

Modern Wheat

Before we discuss wheat, we must first establish what we mean by wheat. Wheat today is radically different than it was sixty years ago and different than its pre-historical ancestors. Wheat was one of the first plants humans cultivated and farmed, directly leading to the foundation of cities and civilization. As humans began to get better at farming, they were able to create more hearty and plentiful strains of the grains such as einkorn or emmer wheat that persisted largely unchanged for thousands of years until the 20th century. Wheat and bread was an integral part of the ancient diet and the most common and abundant food sources throughout history.

With so many people eating wheat throughout history, what's the problem with it today?

The answer is that wheat today is so vastly different to ancient wheat that it is almost unrecognizable in cultivation, processing, taste and texture, and most importantly, biochemical composition.

Modern wheat did not evolve naturally, nor was it developed through gradual cross breeding; it was purposefully developed through countless rounds of hybridization and intense amounts of breeding activity and trial and error within a very short period of time.

The world population approximately doubled between 1900 and 1950 and world hunger was a major concern. Many people attempted to find a way to combat the impending worldwide famine, but none made as much progress as Dr. Norman Borlaug. Dr. Borlaug received a doctorate in plant pathology and genetics and went to the International Maize and Wheat Improvement Center in Mexico to begin working on wheat, along with other scientists to increase the yield, lower the production cost, improve the consistency and make it heartier and more resistant to disease. They certainly succeeded and Borlaug introduced his new dwarf wheat strains all over the world. His new wheat was shorter and had more seeds which hung looser from the stalk allowing for easier threshing, or gathering of the wheat, as well as being more resistant to pesticides.

Though Borlaug and his associates certainly achieved their noble objectives and are credited with saving a billion lives from starvation, we're now becoming aware that the methods used to create the new strains of wheat had unintended consequences.

Using advanced hybridization techniques, Borlaug created countless thousands of unique strains, which continued to be crossbred with their parent strains, other wheat strains or other types of grass. While the alterations were working towards goals like shorter more manageable wheat, the crossbreeding process inevitably created changes outside the scientist's control.

Unlike complex creatures, wheat plants have the ability to retain the sum of the genes from their predecessors. This additive accumulation means that modern wheat can have up to 124,000 genes[5] (compared to 20,000 contained in the human genome), and what's more, it has shown that up to 5% of the proteins expressed in hybrid wheat offspring are found in neither parent[6]. This presents a fundamental challenge to the belief that the composition of hybridized wheat can be predicted from the parent strains

Unlike hybridization, when genetically modified products (a more precise manipulation of the genome using biotechnology) are identified as being significantly different from their predecessor or containing new genes that their predecessor, national authorities require that the foodstuff undergoes safety testing before being released for human consumption. It's assumed that hybridization can't have malignant effects on the genome, so the hybridized wheat wasn't subject to safety testing. What this research shows is that the line between genetic modification and hybridization is blurred, with common wheat having a vastly different and more complex genetic structure than ancient wheat.

Mass Consumption

Though wheat had been one of the most prevalent food products in the world even before all of the intense changes, the new ease of production and higher yields led to wheat being used on a huge scale never before seen. Wheat has become a part of breakfast, lunch, dinner, dessert and snack time. We supplement stacks of pancakes or simply eat cereal for breakfast, enjoy sandwiches for lunch and eat pasta for dinner. When we think about some of the most convenient tasty foods like croissants, doughnuts, crackers and pretzels, they are made with wheat. Things we wouldn't think of like salad dressings, hot dogs, candy and even lipstick can contain wheat or wheat products like gluten.

Modern wheat also has more total gluten proteins and

a much wider variety of these volatile proteins. Gluten is a protein in wheat that gives it pliability, allowing it to be stretched into a pizza or twisted into a pastry. Ancient wheat had far less gluten and less varieties of gluten and while still pliable, would quickly crumble if you were to try to make a croissant. Gluten is a major culprit for the cause of wheat induced health problems and many issues stemming from wheat are caused by the mutated product rather than ancient wheat. Though emmer, einkorn and other ancient wheat contain gluten and have very similar carbohydrate structures, they were present in lower amounts and with lower variety than modern wheat, and those who are allergic or have a sensitivity to gluten have shown fewer problems after consuming ancient wheat. However, we now see that wheat in general, ancient or modern, can harm your body, modern wheat has many more known and unknown mutations that can wreak havoc on the body.

Heath Easton

WHEAT AND THE GUT

By far the most known problem among the host of damaging effects of wheat are gut disorders, celiac disease, gluten sensitivities and wheat allergies. Celiac disease is classified as an autoimmune disorder of the intestine where the presence of certain gluten proteins (mainly gliadin proteins) trigger the creation of enzymes which the body treats as invaders and attacks the gluten as well as the intestine and its enzymes. The body attacks the gluten and the intestine to such a degree that it becomes inflamed and loses its integrity.

The villi, which line the inner ring of the intestine, are responsible for the proper absorption of nutrients. These villi are the first to be damaged and broken down by the body's immune response and the villi begin failing to properly absorb some nutrients while gluten and other wheat proteins can permeate the inner barriers and gain access to the bloodstream. The body reacts with antibodies against the wheat proteins, as well as against components of the compromised intestinal wall and the contents of the gut like bacteria and food molecules.

If gone unchecked, the body's immune response can destroy whole sections of the small intestine and many other areas of the body can be affected as the harmful proteins and antibodies collide throughout the bloodstream.

The intestine is a large and hugely important organ, and this intestinal damage causes the most common symptoms of celiac disease. Diarrhea and cramping from the actual immune response, along with weight loss or failure to grow/ failure to thrive, as seen in children, are common symptoms. The weight loss often comes from malabsorption of food, but can also occur by an aversion to eating, as it becomes too painful. Continued wheat ingestion can scar the intestines, leading to painful ulcers or narrowing of the intestine, possibly leading to abdominal pain, regardless of day to day changes in diet.

But, these symptoms seem benign when compared to other associated effects of celiac disease. Along with direct symptoms, celiac disease, gluten sensitivity and wheat allergies can be associated with many other problems and put you at risk from a whole host of diseases. The disease commonly associated is type 1 or childhood diabetes. Type 1 diabetics are up to twenty times more likely to have or develop celiac disease later in life. The liver can be affected as a blood filtering organ seeing a lot of damage from the glutens and their antibodies. Scarring of the liver can be seen in some patients and an increased risk of cancer is present in those with any level of gluten intolerance[7]. The full list of conditions associated with celiac is mind boggling, including:

- Huntington's
- Non-Hodgkin's lymphoma
- Hypothyroidism
- Lupus
- Vitiligo
- Narcolepsy
- Schizophrenia
- Autism
- Depression
- Porphyria
- Infertility

- Type 1 Diabetes
- Multiple Sclerosis
- Rheumatoid Arthritis

Not only is a disease that is chronically under-diagnosed (it's estimated that only 10-15% of celiac sufferers in the USA know that they have it), but it also appears to be on the rise. Separate studies from the USA and Finland show that in test groups, celiac is four times as prevalent as it was 40 years ago, and twice as prevalent as it was 20 years ago[8].

But I'm not Celiac ...

It would be wrong to suggest the majority of the population who don't have full blown celiac are safe from the damaging effects of wheat and gluten, however. Not only do we now have evidence that non-celiac gluten sensitivity exists from a number of research papers[9] (aside from countless anecdotal accounts), but the process by which gluten invokes an immune response in everyone has been discovered.

Haptoglobin-2, also known as zonulin, discovered in 2000, is a protein that controls the tight junctions between intestinal cells, creating 'leakiness' in the gut. Zonulin is triggered as an adaptive response to certain bacteria, but it has been found that gliadin (a gluten protein) mimics the effect of these bacteria and also triggers zonulin to increase gut leakiness.

This 'gut leakiness' makes the intestine more permeable, allowing the contents of the gut uninhibited entry into the body. The intestine is not supposed to be freely permeable and when the contents of the intestine find their way into the bloodstream, the body reacts with an inflammatory immune response.

Celiac is an autoimmune condition wherein the immune system attacks the body's own tissues, but with intestinal permeability, the immune attacks are directed solely against components of the diet that pass unwanted through the gut. Damage to the intestine may be less persistent or intense, but many of the same symptoms can exist and the immune and inflammatory response is similarly invoked, caused by the same pathogen – gluten.

Dr Fasano, who discovered zonulin, has found that the gut leakiness effect of gliadin occurs in everybody, not just celiacs. Although the effect is more intense and prolonged for those with celiac (about fivefold), the same mechanism of action occurs in everyone[10].

Autoimmune disease and inflammation have many underlying serious conditions like Crohn's disease, diabetes, celiac and others discussed in this book, and it's thought the gliadian-zonulin-intestinal leakiness mechanism could be a factor in these conditions. There are at least 80 different autoimmune conditions that affect humans, who are the only species that have the modified gene for zonulin. Surprisingly, other primates (who don't have this gene), don't experience autoimmune diseases.

It is important to note that many suffering from some form of gluten sensitivity may not present painful or outwardly noticeable symptoms. Even if the intestine is damaged, it is possible to be present without noticeable side effects. Without the tell-tale symptoms, wheat can infiltrate your bloodstream and cause all kinds of havoc.

Even more troublesome is that standard lab tests may not reveal gluten sensitivity. A recent study looking at children with type 1 diabetes found that a significant number of them had celiac. Of these children, some had a positive antibody test for celiac, but many showed negative results on both the common blood test for celiac and on an intestinal biopsy[11]. So, medical professionals would have ruled out the influence of gluten in their condition.

The study suggested that most of the kids would go on to develop celiac. What this tells us is gut damage can present few symptoms but still lead to autoimmunity. Autoimmunity can and will progress to other problems, but doctors will rule it out, particularly in the presence of a negative blood test.

Can you afford to gamble with your health? Can you afford to wait until the general medical consensus catches up with what the research suggests? Considering the increasing prevalence and endemic under diagnosis, gluten sensitivity links to much more serious conditions. The fact that gluten can cause a similar autoimmune response in everyone should cause us to pause and reflect on the wisdom of recommending this food as part of a balanced diet.

Heath Easton

WHEAT AND OBESITY

Obesity is one of the biggest killers in the western world. Obesity related illness, including heart disease; stroke and diabetes greatly surpass cancers as the leading cause of death in America and most of the rest of the world. Obesity is linked to countless ailments from joint problems to stroke and obesity is even associated with lowering IQs.

What has been the prevalent belief in American nutritional wisdom is that fats, such as milk and animal fat directly cause body fat. This correlation can certainly be appealing as it is easy to say that eating fat makes you fat, but it is not nearly that simple. Not all fat is created equal and animal fats may actually be some of the healthiest fats you can eat; while avoiding fats by eating carbohydrates promotes the accumulation of body fat.

When you see a big label on a favorite food, declaring it low fat or fat free you might think it is a guilt free indulgence. The truth is that foods advertising less fat often compensate by adding more sugar or are simple carbohydrate foods like crackers or bagels. As grains continue to form the base of the nutritional pyramid, they are still one of the most consumed types of food with carbohydrates, often comprising nearly 80% or more of the daily diet. This amount of grain and wheat in particular, has a profound effect on body fat storage.

As we know, wheat causes larger blood sugar spikes than actual sugar, which in turn prompts the release of insulin from the pancreas. Insulin signals the body's cells to accept glucose, which is the main fuel for every cell in the body. When we have excess blood sugar, however, insulin's job is to convert it to fat and store it in the body.

This can be fat under the skin (subcutaneous fat), around the thighs, buttocks or arms, but consistent spikes in blood sugar can also (for unknown reasons) lead to fat deposits around the centre of the body in between the internal organs, often resulting in what used to be called a beer belly, but should now be more appropriately referred to as a wheat belly.

Most people think of fat as just extra padding, with a protruding belly simply equating to a little extra weight that you have to lug around. Few people might be aware this intra-organ fat – known as visceral fat - can cause hormonal changes in your body, producing estrogen and other hormones and causing a great deal of inflammation among many other adverse effects.

While subcutaneous fat mainly serves as energy storage and has limited adverse effects, visceral abdominal fat harms the body in many ways. A major correlation between diabetes and increased waistline size has been thoroughly researched and conversely a decrease of waistline size in obese patients reduces or can even eliminate many of the symptoms of type 2 diabetes. This correlation certainly involves the fact that high blood sugars over time can lead to diabetes while simultaneously leading to the creation and storage of more visceral fat. However, the improvements seen with just a reduction of visceral fat in diabetic patients show that the fat itself, worsens the effects of diabetes. When a sufficient amount of visceral fat accumulates, it has an inflammatory response that cause many cells to respond less to insulin leading to a proportionally greater amount of insulin to be released by the pancreas which in turn results in more creation of visceral fat and strains the pancreas leading to a greater likelihood of developing type 2 diabetes.

Visceral fat is unique in that it produces a variety of hormones which can throw your body way out of its natural rhythm. A modest amount of visceral fat produces the fullness hormone leptin as well as adiponectin, which works to regulate insulin and energy levels. While these hormones are great to have to maintain a proper diet, an abundance of visceral fat alters the way these hormones are released, usually correlating to less of these good hormones with the more visceral fat gained.

If you are a man, wheat can not only give you a protruding belly, it can give you full male breasts as well. Visceral fat also produces estrogen, and while females can usually handle an extra dose of estrogen, it can wreak havoc on a man's hormonal balance. Not only does estrogen contribute to forming male breasts (moobs – not a good look), but in excess levels it can increase your risk for heart disease and prostate cancer and further increase body fat. Once excessive visceral fat is accrued, it causes a series of chain reactions from increased insulin resistance to lower fullness hormones and more weight gain hormones. It is a vicious cycle, but can be slowed and reversed by eliminating the biggest culprit: carbohydrate foods like wheat.

Heath Easton

WHEAT AND DIABETES

While it has been mentioned multiple times above it deserves to be mentioned again; wheat increases you blood sugar as much or more than an equivalent amount of regular cola, candy or table sugar. Diabetes continues to increase with nearly half of Americans being diabetic or pre-diabetic[12]. It is an explosion of about a 15-20% over the past thirty years. There is a correlation between modern wheat cementing its place in the diet as well as the aversion of traditional fat foods such as meat and butter and replacing those calories with empty carbohydrates. While many people know that excessive consumption of junk food such as soda and candy and physical inactivity can be risk factors for developing type 2 diabetes, it is not widely known how much of an impact wheat, even whole wheat, has on developing diabetes and worsening the symptoms of diabetics.

The development of diabetes is simple in theory, but can be quite complex as it develops. When blood sugars spike, it takes a moderate toll on the pancreas, which not only produces a great deal of insulin, but also increases the amount of insulin secreting cells known as beta cells. The problem with large spike in blood sugar is that the excess glucose can damage the beta cells. In combination with beta cell damage from triglycerides formed by glucose, this causes the pancreas to have difficulty producing enough insulin to keep up with the levels of glucose in the blood. When the pancreas is not able to manage blood sugar, we have a diagnosis of diabetes.

High amounts of visceral fat compound the problem, leading to inflammation and causing muscle and liver cells to be resistant to insulin producing even more insulin with less and less efficiency of distributing the blood sugar.

So, we have established that diabetes is caused by repeated exposure to high glycemic foods such as wheat and is worsened by visceral fat. This is a terrible, chronic disease that not only reduces the average life expectancy by eight years, but also incurs added medical expenses of hundreds of thousands of dollars over the course of your life. It is one of the top ten causes of death and is rising fast enough to be one of the top three killers within a decade or two.

As obesity correlates so strongly with the onset and progression of diabetes as well as heart disease, treatments often involve a fat restricted fat diet in addition a large proportion of whole grains. The problem with these methods is that they are not addressing the cause of the damage: high blood sugar.

Drastically reducing carbohydrate consumption to 10% or lower has proven to be incredibly effective at reducing and often eliminating the symptoms and underlying causes of diabetes. As high blood sugar prompts insulin production, damages beta cells, and creates more visceral fat, eliminating occurrences of high blood sugar can completely halt the progression of diabetes and allow the body to heal itself. The first step is the reduction of visceral fat, which allows cells to be much more receptive to insulin. Decreased blood sugar spikes then began to prompt less and less insulin production from the pancreas and it can attempt to heal itself and the remaining functioning beta cells. In many cases, medications, including insulin shots can be reduced or eliminated and simple blood monitoring and dietary adjustments are all that's needed.

A study by Temple University reduced the carbohydrate intake of obese diabetics by only allowing 21 grams per day. This led to an average loss of 3.6 pounds and saw a 75% improvement in insulin response, the ability of the pancreas to secrete enough insulin. In a few cases, the damage to the pancreas is too extensive and it is simply unable to handle even small amounts of glucose. Even in these cases symptoms improve greatly and management became much easier. Diabetes is a chronic and often fatal disease that can be almost entirely reduced if we eliminate blood sugar spiking wheat and other carbohydrates. It really is as simple as that.

GRAINS ON THE BRAIN

We now know how wheat can jack up your blood sugar and cause whole body immune responses that can damage almost any part of your body. But, you might be surprised that it can have neurological effects. Believe it or not, there are multiple brain and nerve conditions that are brought on, or severely worsened, by wheat and gluten. Some are a gradual onset, meaning they may not even be noticed until years later after the damage is done, some are life-threatening. While many of the conditions are so seemingly unrelated to diet that wheat has only recently been considered as a factor.

Wheat has recently been associated with a variety of mental conditions largely because wheat free diets have suddenly halted or reversed several symptoms of various neurological problems. It's quite an announcement to say that psychiatric hospitals would be much better places if wheat was restricted or eliminated. However, research suggests wheat can worsen some psychiatric illness, such as schizophrenia, autism and depression. This seems quite far-fetched as schizophrenia is usually a fairly progressive disease, making it difficult to pin on normal dietary habits. Also, small studies in psychiatric hospitals have shown that symptoms of schizophrenia drastically improved on a gluten-free diet.

Dr. F. Curtis Dohan, a prolific medical researcher, was one of the first to make the connection. While serving as a flight surgeon during WWII, Dohan observed that food shortages, which limited the amount of bread available, also lowered the amount of hospitalizations for schizophrenic symptoms. Later, Dohan observed that the level of schizophrenia was low in New Guinea as they ate a Palaeolithic-type diet. As modern food, including wheat, entered the diet, schizophrenia became 65 times more common. Finally, Dohan was able to test wheat with schizophrenia directly. While working at a veteran's hospital in Philadelphia Dr. Dohan and his team abruptly removed all wheat products from schizophrenic patients. This resulted in both a significant reduction of hallucinations and increased patients' attachment to reality over the course of only a few weeks. Once wheat products were reintroduced the symptoms increased.

Autism is another such condition in which the links are beginning to appear between gut health, diet and symptoms. Since 1995, autism alone has gone from a rate of 1/3300 children to 1/88 children[13]. There is no scientifically backed cure to autism and the causes and risk factors associated with the condition are still unclear, but small studies[14] and anecdotal evidence suggest a link between the severity of symptoms and gluten intake and gut health. Removal of gluten from the diet has shown improvements in the symptoms of autistic children[15].

New research is in progress; however, it seems clear that there are also strong ties between wheat and cerebral ataxia, with a subset even known as gluten ataxia. Ataxia is characterized predominantly by a loss of balance and coordination. Ataxia can progress from simple stumbling and difficulty with hand eye coordination to having difficulty standing straight and using your arms and hands to complete simple tasks like eating or brushing your teeth.

Much of this is an assumed side effect of age, but evidence suggests that a lifelong indulgence in harmful wheat products is a factor for some. Those with celiac disease show an increased likelihood of developing ataxia, while close to half of those who have otherwise unexplained ataxia show some sort of wheat or gluten intolerance.

A recent study even found that a gluten-free diet led to a remission in symptoms of depression in patients with non-celiac gluten sensitivity[16]. It's also worth pointing out that some studies show that even when gluten worsens neurological symptoms, gastro-intestinal symptoms may not worsen or may even be completely absent. One study[17] showed that 13% of patients with gluten ataxia had no GI symptoms. Another study[18] found that while isolated gluten added to a gluten-free diet did not worsen GI symptoms, it did increase symptoms of depression in a group of patients with self-reported non-celiac gluten sensitivity.

One might also be surprised to learn that finally ousting wheat could prove to be as difficult as quitting smoking, not only because those morning doughnuts are just that tasty, but because wheat has the same addictive chemical impacts on the brain that many addictive drugs have.

Institute of Health investigators found that when gliadin (a component of gluten) is digested, it's broken down into a potent opiate-like substance, which they dubbed 'exorphins'[19]. In those with damaged brains this morphine like high causes an already overactive brain to go into overdrive. Studies using the opiate blocking drug naloxone have shown that it also blocks the similar brain altering effects of the broken down gluten peptides. Giving naloxone to schizophrenics has improved their symptoms similar to removing wheat. So wheat has peptides that bind with the brain's morphine receptor, and while they certainly do not give the intense high of most opiate drugs, they do trigger the brains reward center.

Constant triggering of the reward center stimulates appetite and will eventually result in withdrawal when wheat is eliminated with very similar effects as withdrawing from some opiates or other addictive substances. A study at the Psychiatric institute of South Carolina showed that normal diet wheat eaters consumed an average of 28% less calories when given the opiate blocking drug naloxone which blocked the addictive appetite stimulating effect of wheat. Once the withdrawal period is over many people have little difficulty sticking to a wheat free diet, although going through withdraw is a difficult hurdle for many.

WHEAT AND HEART DISEASE

Whole wheat has, in the past few decades, been touted to be a heart healthy whole grain. An important part of the diet to lower cholesterol and improve heart health, wheat was essential while animal fats were demonized and almost certainly caused all manner of heart disease. The problem is that the advice to cut fats from the diet in favour of whole grains hasn't yielded the reduction in heart disease that the theories predicted. Most famously exemplified the "Eisenhower Paradox" whereby President Dwight Eisenhower practically renounced all fatty foods from his diet in an attempt to reduce his cholesterol levels following a heart attack aged 64. Despite the adaption's to his diet at the suggestion of his doctors, his cholesterol continued to rise and he suffered 6 more heart attacks over the next 14 years, eventually succumbing in 1969.

While national authorities have the best interests of their public at heart (pun intended,) they don't always get it right when it comes to dietary recommendations. Authors like a Gary Taubes have done a great job of bringing the dietary health debate into the public domain and pointing out that governments don't necessarily always come to the right conclusions in the domain of health. While a solitary chapter isn't sufficient to fully explore all sides of the theories around heart disease it's worth noting the potential link between wheat and heart disease

Whilst dietary fat has long being implicated as the leading cause of heart disease, blood sugar and insulin spikes have recently been considered as a more likely cause. This means sugary and high carb foods are implicated, including wheat – which as we know, have a higher glycemic index than pure table sugar

The most damaging aspect of wheat on the heart is the type of fat it creates in the body. This last sentence might cause some people to pause as whole grains are supposed to be cholesterol free and have 'heart healthy' fiber. The problem lies not with what initially goes into our bodies but what wheat makes our bodies do. The high blood sugar spike caused by wheat causes the abundance of insulin to create energy dense triglycerides and very low density lipoproteins known as cholesterol. There are many types of cholesterol and not all are bad. HDL, high density lipoproteins, are good for you and help balance out the LDL cholesterol which comes in large and small varieties. A complex set of reactions after high blood sugar spikes causes the liver to produce triglycerides and VLDL which can from great quantities of small LDL cholesterol. Small LDL is the worst as its name implies, it is small. This allows it to get into smaller vessels and may allow greater build-ups of cholesterol in dangerous spots. Small LDL is also more prone to harmful oxidation which can cause a dangerous hardening of the arteries. VLDL and large and small LDL cholesterol are still being researched but there is strong, correlating evidence that small LDL particles drastically increase the risk of heart disease and heart attacks in particular. Wheat in particular has been shown to increase the small LDL cholesterol far more than many other carbohydrates, including a 60% increase when compared to an oat diet[20].

Aside from the deadly specific small LDL particles created by wheat, there are a few other negative effects on the heart caused by wheat. Visceral fat created by wheat consumption takes up residence around the major organs including the heart. An excess of this fat causes inflammation of the tissues around it while also becoming inflamed itself. This inflammation can weaken the vessels around the heart while the amount of fat can put added stress on the cardiac muscles themselves. As mentioned above, the body often attacks components of wheat gluten as it gains access to the bloodstream causing autoimmune responses and inflammation in all areas of the body and the heart is no exception. Most common symptom of this autoimmune response is damage or a hardening of the vessels. Constant high blood sugars, whether full blown diabetes or just continued consumption of high glycemic foods can cause the glucose to deteriorate the inner lining and arteries around the heart, one of the reasons diabetics have such a higher risk for heart disease.

What is amazing is that once again a wheat free/reduced carbohydrate diet shows drastic improvements to heart health. Even with continued consumption of butter and other animal fats LDL cholesterol and total fat can be greatly reduced with low carb diets[21]. As heart disease is one of the leading causes of death today, it seems that a worldwide reduction of wheat consumption – creating a reduction in overall carbohydrate consumption - could save many lives. But unfortunately far too many people are still under the impression that whole wheat will keep them heart healthy and awareness has yet to spread despite more studies pointing to high fat creation and heart disease risks of wheat.

Heath Easton

WHEAT AND ACNE

Acne is the scourge of the teenager, one of the most embarrassing phases of growing up. Not only is it very common, it tends to be a persistent problem and is difficult to control. It would be wrong to suggest this is only an adult problem, however, with large amounts of people experiencing adult acne.

	Prevelance of Acne	
Age (Years)	Women	Men
20-29	50.9%	42.5%
30-39	35.2%	20.1%
40-49	26.3%	12.0%
50+	15.3%	7.3%

Source: *The prevalence of acne in adults 20 years and older*, Collier, Harper et al, Journal of the American Academy of Dermatology, 2008

Countless products are specifically made to treat acne and many doctors prescribe harsh medications, whilst there are countless products used to cover up that acne after all else fails. While many people acknowledge that food can play a large role in the formation of acne few people would ever suspect that healthy whole wheat could possibly be a problem. Many people blame high fat, greasy diets with saturated fats and suggest increased whole-grain intake to combat the problem, when in reality wheat and gluten can make acne worse.

As we've learned, wheat cause blood sugar spikes similar to sugary soft drinks, which in turn increases insulin production. A link between insulin and acne has emerged over the last few years, for example one study showed that college students who were administered a low-glycemic index diet showed close to a 25% reduction of acne, while those who eliminated or nearly eliminated carbohydrates saw closer to 50% reduction of acne[22]. The diets of populations for which acne is completely absent are also notably low glycemic-index – the Kivatan Islanders, the Okinawans, the Inuit and the Peruvian Indians.

One of the side effects of insulin is the creation of a

hormone known as insulin-like growth factor (IGF-1). This growth factor will make the skin produce more cells rapidly and increases hair follicle growth. It has also been found to be a big player in acne as it prompts the sebaceous cells to secrete more sebum[23]. Sebum is a protective body oil essential in small quantities to preserve skin but in large amounts will give the skin an oily covering which often clogs pores and promotes acne.

Acne is classed as a low-level inflammatory condition. Inflammation has been shown to play a huge role in acne, with anti-inflammatory foods and medications easing symptoms and inflammation-causing foods doing the opposite[24]. It follows that since wheat and grain consumption promote inflammation through the action of glutens and their antibodies[25], consumption of wheat and grains also promote acne. As mentioned, wheat can also be a causative factor in visceral fat, which also has an inflammatory effect on the body.

Aside from acne there are a wide range of skin rashes that are directly or indirectly related to wheat consumption. Dermatitis herpetiformis is a particular inflammation of the skin that looks similar to a herpes infection though is not actually caused by the herpes virus. This is one of the few rashes that can be directly tied to wheat and can present at any time though more commonly in the 20-30 age range. The only proven cure aside from dangerous drugs is to simply eliminate wheat. Symptoms improve and disappear within days or sometimes months in severe cases. It is crazy to think that a painfully itchy rash that looks a lot like a STD can be caused by something as simple as cereal in the morning, but avoiding it is as simple as avoiding wheat.

Though acne and Dermatitis herpetiformis are the two most common skin problems associated with wheat, there are many more conditions:

● The inflammation effect of wheat can cause skin inflammation and swelling of the small blood vessels on the skin known as cutaneous vasculitis.

● Psoriasis, a common problem involving an itchy red, scaly and flaky rash found often on the scalp can see improvement on a wheat free diet[26].

● Vitiligo, the absence of pigment or bleaching appearance on patches of skin often seen on the hands is often permanent but anecdotal reports indicate that it but can slow significantly with a reduction of wheat.

These and many other rashes can range from minor irritations to painful or utter humiliating scourges of the skin that can destroy your health and ruin your self-confidence and psyche. All can be helped or at least better managed with elimination of wheat and gluten. Any number of skin care products can claim to target the root cause of acne but the only sure-fire way to reduce acne is improve whole body health, and one of the easiest ways to do that is to eliminate gluten, wheat, and high glycemic carbohydrates.

Heath Easton

WHEAT'S AGING EFFECT

Aging is a natural, inevitable part of life. Some do it gracefully; others fight it cosmetically or with surgery, while some simply age horribly. Many people link a rough lifestyle, overindulgence in drink, late nights and smoking with premature aging while aging gracefully means eating healthy and taking care of your body. Few people would ever guess that wheat can cause premature aging to a far greater degree than many other foods. Wrinkles and white hair are not the only signs of aging; damaged eyes, and decreased function of internal organs and unique stiffening of blood vessels eventually get to everyone, though they get to some people decades sooner.

Uncovering the processes of aging has proven to be quite difficult, even though there are several scientists solely dedicated to better understanding how aging works. It is difficult to predict when someone will develop wrinkles or when their heart will finally start to give out. Some scientists seem to have found at least part of the answer. The presence of substances known as advanced glycation end-products, abbreviated as AGE, often directly correlate with common signs of ageing. In essence, the more AGEs you have, the higher your body's age, otherwise referred to as your physiological age. AGE are cells in which glucose combines with proteins which make cells less flexible and more prone to irreversible damage. AGEs form in the body due to high blood sugar and when wheat is habitually consumed it gives the body a semi-constant source of glucose to form AGE. The development of diabetes further ensures a steady source of blood glucose.

AGE affect aging in many ways, primarily because the glucose combination can occur in virtually every cell in the body but are most prevalent in a few key areas and slowly, but steadily cause often irreversible damage. The stiff and often damaged cells affected by AGE often lose the ability to function normally in whichever system they were part of. Skin cells cannot hold together as well, individual kidney cells lose their ability to filter blood and brain cells lose their ability to properly signal each other. The exact mechanisms of how AGE damages the body are unknown or largely unproven. However, in almost all cases of age related organ failure and brain problems such as dementia, AGEs were found in higher quantities than normal. While AGE can be formed outside the body in some meats and cigarettes, and acquisition of AGE is unavoidable no matter the diet, foods such as wheat greatly increase their production.

Heath Easton

YOUR WHEATECTOMY

So, we've learned about the unusual development of modern wheat and learned about a few of its effects on the body. We know that through the action of some of the proteins in wheat like gluten and through wheat's effect on blood sugar, it is connected with a mind-boggling array of health conditions. The next question then is, how should I use this information? How does it affect me?

It's clear from looking at the widespread damage wheat and gluten exert on the body and the sheer number of health conditions that have been linked to wheat and gluten that there's only one solution for optimum health and longevity – the removal of wheat and gluten from the diet.

A wheat-free diet is a great start, and I recommend taking any action over doing nothing at all. But, in order to avoid the damaging effect of gluten on the body a gluten-free diet is best, which includes things like spelt, rye, oats, barley and other grains. It might sound intimidating to stop eating what has become such a prolific foodstuff from your diet, but don't worry, I'm here to help you achieve the gluten-free healthy lifestyle that many have already achieved. So let's get down to the nitty gritty.

I see two approaches commonly used when approaching a wheatectomy:

- **The piecemeal approach** – a tapering diet where gluten products are removed from routine over time. For example, you might start removing gluten from breakfast, lunch, and then dinner over the course of a few weeks, or only eat gluten products at the weekend for a while.

- **All at once** – Cutting out gluten in all its forms, without exception.

I recommend a complete removal from the diet. While cutting down on gluten will undoubtedly have benefits for everyone, the only way observe how your body reacts to gluten and to gauge the benefits that a gluten-free diet can have on your heath and body are to completely exclude them.

If ditching the gluten products sounds horrific or overwhelming to you or you're not convinced that it's worth it, remember than you can always go back to your old diet (30 days or so is recommended) if the experiment doesn't yield the results you expected (I'm confident it will – most people feel great after being gluten-free a few weeks).

So, give yourself pat yourself a pat on the back for making it this far, take a deep breath, then roll up your sleeves and gird up your loins for action. Check out these top tips for tackling your new gluten-free lifestyle

Top Tips For Going Gluten Free

1. Focus on what you can have – not what you can't have. Millions of people are gluten-free and there's an abundance of recipes and support online.

2. Don't aim for endless amounts of variation initially or you'll end up overwhelming yourself. Focus on mastering a few core meals and incorporating them

into your weekly routine before experimenting with new foods and meals. Variety is overrated, at least in the beginning.

3. Keep it simple. Focus on whole foods like meat, eggs, fish, vegetables, fruits and nuts. Avoid the temptation to replace all your favourite grain foods with pre-packaged gluten-free substitutes. In many cases they're absent of gluten but are still highly processed, low in nutritional value and high in other toxins.

4. Take time to congratulate yourself on taking these steps to increase your health and happiness. One day at a time – you can do this!

5. Learn a few recipes for naturally gluten-free alternatives to your favorite gluten foods – check out the recipes below for zucchini noodles, mushroom burger buns, nori wraps and grain-free porridge for good alternatives to pasta, sandwiches and porridge.

6. Consider planning some or all of your meals in advance. This means you can are less likely to default to a convenience food like a sandwich or pasta when you can't decide what to eat. Visit here to get a meal

planner to help with this.

7. Look out for hidden sources of gluten like some alcohols (e.g. beer) and certain sauces (e.g. béchamel). Check out the cheat sheet here for a breakdown of what to look out for. Cut it out and stick it up inside your kitchen cupboard for quick reference.

8. You may feel off the first few days being gluten-free – this is your body's reaction to removing wheat (due to its addictive properties, as we've discussed) and you'll bounce back after a few days. You may even feel horrendous during this cold turkey phase – just remember it's because of years of wheat abuse and you'll feel a million times better once you're through to the other side.

9. Maintaining a gluten-free diet is perfectly possible in most restaurants and in many, it's a breeze. Get used to asking the waiter if a dish contains gluten if you're not sure and be prepared to ask them to sub out bread for extra veggies or salad.

10. Not being prepared is your enemy, especially when combined with hunger. Consider keeping some emergency snacks in your desk or car for when hunger strikes and the only other option is a subway –

e.g. nuts, seeds, jars of olives of olives or artichokes, jerky or biltong, etc.

RECIPES

BREAKFAST

Greek Yoghurt and Fruit

Prep time: 2 minutes
Servings: 1

Ingredients
1 pot natural Greek yoghurt or goat yoghurt
A couple of handfuls of fresh berries or sliced fruit
1 tsp natural honey
Optional: Crushed or flaked nuts

Instructions
- Pour your chosen selection of fruit, berries and nuts into the yoghurt. Drizzle with honey, and eat.

Grain-Free Coconut Porridge

Prep time: 10 minutes
Cooking time: 10 minutes
Servings: 1

Ingredients

2 Tbsp of almond butter
¼ cup of coconut, shredded
6 Tbsp of warm water or coconut milk (full-fat)
¼ tsp of vanilla extract
½ tsp of cinnamon
1 tsp of raw honey or maple syrup (melted)

Instructions

- In a small mixing bowl, combine almond butter, shredded coconut, water or coconut milk, vanilla extract, cinnamon and honey or maple syrup. Stir to combine.

- Transfer mixture into a saucepan and simmer over low heat until heated through.

Grain-Free Vanilla Almond Sponge Bread

Prep time: 10 minutes
Cooking time: 40 minutes
Servings: 6

Ingredients

6 eggs
¼ pod of vanilla beans, seeds scraped
1 tsp of vanilla extract
2 Tbsp of butter (melted)
2 Tbsp of coconut milk (full-fat)
¼ cup of coconut flour
Pinch of nutmeg
Pinch of sea salt
½ tsp of baking soda
2 Tbsp of almonds, sliced

Instructions

- Preheat oven to 350°F/180°C. Line a 9x9-inch baking dish with parchment paper.
- In a large mixing bowl, whisk eggs, butter and coconut milk.
- Add in sifted flour, nutmeg, salt and baking soda and continue whisking until well combined.
- Transfer the mixture into the prepared baking dish.
- Sprinkle almond slices on top and bake for 40

minutes or until the edges are brown or a toothpick inserted in center comes out clean.

GrainFreeNola with Dried Strawberries

Prep time: 20 minutes

Cooking time: 3 hours (mostly hands off)

Servings: 10-12

Ingredients

2 ½ cups of raw almonds

2 cups of macadamia nuts

1 ½ cups of coconut flakes

10 medium strawberries

6 dried apricots, finely diced

2/3 cup of dried cranberries

2/3 cup of dried Goji berries

2/3 cup of Chia seeds

Instructions

- Preparing oven dried strawberries takes a lot of time. To do this, you need to wash fresh strawberries then pat them dry and sliced lengthwise. Slice each strawberry into 6 slices.

- Preheat the oven to the lowest heat settings possible, 165°F/75°C.

- Use a rack or tray that has holes and spread the strawberry slices so the hot air can circulate under them.

- Place strawberries in oven and dry/bake for 2 to 3

hours. After 2 hours of baking time, carefully turn the strawberry slices over.

- Remove strawberries from the oven and let it cool, and increase the heat up to 300°F/150°C.

- Roast almonds and macadamia nuts in a large baking tray for 10 minutes, stirring every 2 minutes or until golden brown and have a nice toasted smell (you need to stir the nuts frequently towards the end of the roasting period.)

- Transfer nuts to a bowl and set aside to cool.

- In the same baking pan, roast the coconut flakes for 5 minutes or until golden brown. Always check on them, stirring halfway through.

- Grind the nuts coarsely using a food processor.

- In a large bowl, combine nuts, coconut flakes, apricots, strawberries, cranberries, Goji berries and Chia seeds. Mix well and let it cool down completely.

- Store in an airtight container for a few weeks, if not gobbled up quickly.

Sweet Potato Rosti with Smoked Salmon and Lemon

Prep time: 15 minutes

Cooking time: 10 minutes

Servings: 2

Ingredients

½ large sweet potato, peeled

1 egg

1 Lebanese cucumber

¼ white onion, peeled

5.5oz smoked salmon

1 lemon or lime

Black pepper

Sea salt

1 Tbsp of ghee (clarified butter)

1 tsp of olive oil

Optional: Fresh dill to garnish

Instructions

- Grate the sweet potatoes and add in 1 whole egg. Season with ½ tsp sea salt and a pinch of cracked black pepper.

- Heat 1 Tbsp of ghee in a skillet and place the potato mix to the center of the skillet and flatten with spatula to about 70mm.

- Lower the heat to medium and fry, covered for 5 minutes.
- Gently flip the pancake and put a large plate face down on top of the skillet and turn upside down, to help the pancake to transfer to a plate cooked side up.
- Melt another ½ tsp of ghee in a skillet and slide the pancake back into the pan.
- Cook, uncovered for about 3 minutes on low heat; then turn up the heat to medium and cook for further 4 minutes.
- Meanwhile, peel cucumber and slice into long strips. Thinly slice the onion.
- Transfer pancake to a large serving platter. Spread 1 Tbsp of mayonnaise, then top with salmon slices, cucumber strips and onion slices.
- Drizzle on top with lime or lemon juice and olive oil and season with some black pepper.
- Garnish with fresh dill.

Breakfast Pumpkin Pancakes

Prep time: 10 minutes
Cooking time: 20 minutes
Servings: 8 small pancakes or 2 servings

Ingredients
4 eggs
½ cup of canned pumpkin
1 tsp of pure vanilla extract
2 Tbsp of pure maple syrup (optional)
1 tsp of pumpkin pie spice
1 tsp of cinnamon
¼ tsp of baking soda
2 Tbsp of butter or coconut oil (plus extra for pan frying)

Instructions
- In a large mixing bowl, combine the eggs, canned pumpkin, vanilla extract and maple syrup and whisk them together.
- Sift the pumpkin pie spice, cinnamon and baking soda directly on the wet ingredients.
- Heat a small saucepan over medium heat and melt 2 Tbsp of butter.
- Add melted butter to the pancake mixture.
- Heat the skillet and grease lightly with melted butter

or coconut oil.

- Spoon some pancake batter into the skillet, depending to your desired size.

- Cook pancakes until few small bubbles appear on the surface, the turn to flip the other side and cook until light golden in color.

- Serve hot pancakes, topped with a slice of butter and drizzled with maple syrup.

LUNCH

Tuna Nicoise Salad

Prep time: 10 minutes
Cooking time: 20 minutes
Servings: 4

Ingredients

12-15 baby potatoes, unpeeled and thickly sliced
2 Tbsp of olive oil
2 tsp of olive oil
4 eggs
2 Tbsp of capers, rinsed
1.8oz Sun Blush or sun dried tomatoes in oil, finely chopped
½ red onion, thinly sliced
3.5oz baby spinach
2 x cans (~15oz each) yellow fin tuna steak in spring water, drained

Instructions

- Preheat oven to 200°C/fan 180°C/gas 6.
- Season the potatoes with 2 tsp oil and some seasonings.
- Arrange potatoes on a large baking pan and roast, stirring halfway until crisp and golden brown, about 20 minutes.

- Meanwhile, boil the eggs depending on how you liked them cooked.

- Submerge eggs into a bowl of cold water, then peel away the shells and cut each egg in half.

- Whisk the remaining oil in a salad bowl, together with red wine vinegar, capers and chopped tomatoes.

- Stir in the onions, spinach, tuna and potatoes. Toss everything together.

- Garnish salad with boiled eggs and serve immediately.

Greek Salad

Prep time: 10 minutes
Cooking time: 10 minutes
Servings: 8

Ingredients
3 cucumbers, seeded and sliced
1 ½ cups of Feta cheese, crumbled
1 cup of black olives, pitted and sliced
3 cups of Roma tomatoes, diced
1/3 cup of diced, oil packed sun-dried tomatoes (drained, oil reserved)
½ red onion, sliced

Instructions
- In a large salad bowl, combine cucumbers, feta cheese, olives, Roma tomatoes, sun-dried tomatoes, 2 tablespoons reserved sun-dried tomato oil, and red onion. Toss together gently till combined.
- Chill just before serving.

Nori Wraps with 3 Filling Ideas

Prep time: 10 minutes
Cooking time: 5 minutes
Servings: 1

Ingredients

For the Rice-free Nori Rolls
1 sheet Nori seaweed
1-2 small cos lettuce leaves
Tamari (wheat-free) soy sauce, to serve

For the Tuna Sauerkraut Slaw filling
¼ cup of packet slaw mix, undressed
¼ cup of tuna in olive oil, drained and mashed
Small handful of sauerkraut
1 sprig coriander or parsley
Chili powder or pepper, to taste

For the Sprouted Omelette filling
1 egg, free-range or organic preferred
1 Tbsp of mung bean sprouts
2 Tbsp of feta cheese, crumbled

Crunchy Broccoli and Chicken filling

1/3 cup of chicken barbecue, shredded

½ cup of broccoli florets, sliced

1 avocado, diced

chili powder or pepper to taste

Instructions

<u>To make the Rice-free Nori Rolls</u>

- Lay nori sheets on a flat surface and place 2 small cos lettuce leaves starting on the edges nearest you.

- Spoon fillings of your choice and place on top of the leaves.

- Press the ingredients down and fold over the end nearest you, wrapping snugly towards the farthest end.

- Repeat this step with the remaining nori rolls.

- You can cut each rolls or eat whole and serve with tamari soy sauce.

<u>To make the Sprouted Omelette</u>

- In a large bowl, whisk the eggs, sprouts and feta.

- Heat a greased skillet and cook the omellete over medium high heat for 5 to 6 minutes.

Caprese Salad

Prep time: 10 minutes
Cooking time: 10 minutes
Servings: 4-6

Ingredients

3 vine-ripe tomatoes, ¼-inch thick slices
1 lb fresh mozzarella, ¼-inch thick slices
20 to 30 leaves fresh basil (about 1 bunch)
Extra virgin olive oil (for drizzling)
Coarse salt and pepper

Instructions

- Arrange slices of tomatoes and mozzarella alternately in a shallow platter.
- Add a basil leaf between each layer.
- Drizzle extra virgin olive oil over the salad, then sprinkle with coarse salt and pepper to taste

Portabello and Halloumi Burgers

Prep time: 5 minutes
Cooking time: 10 minutes
Servings: 2

Ingredients
4 portabello mushroom caps with stems removed
3 ½ Tbsp of balsamic vinegar
Optional: 2 beef burgers (make sure they're flour-free)
2 Tbsp of oil
2 thin slices of halloumi
2 thick slices tomato
Sea salt and black pepper
A handful of basil leaves

Instructions
- Heat the grill over medium high heat.
- Wash the mushrooms caps and dry with paper towels.
- In a bowl, whisk together balsamic vinegar and olive oil and brush this mixture onto the mushrooms.
- Grill the mushrooms for about 5 minutes on one side until they start to sweat. Flip to grill the other side, about 3 minutes more.
- Meanwhile, cook the burgers to your liking in a

separate pan, on a medium-high heat for about 4 minutes each side for medium-rare.

- When the mushrooms are done, grill halloumi over high heat for about 2 minutes on each side until grill marks form on the cheese and the cheese becomes soft and pliable.

- Season tomato slices with salt and pepper.

- To assemble the burger, use the mushrooms as the buns, the halloumi and burger as the filling and topped with tomato slices and fresh basil leaves.

- Wrap in burger wrapper and serve hot.

Silky Celeriac Soup

Prep time: 10 minutes
Cooking time: 45 minutes
Servings: 4

Ingredients
4 Tbsp butter or coconut oil
4 celery stalks, chopped
1 leek, or 2 shallots, sliced
2 large celeriac roots, peeled and cut into 1/2-inch cubes
1½ quarts water
½ cup heavy cream or coconut milk
Salt and pepper to taste
¼ cup finely chopped fresh parsley

Instructions
- Melt the butter or coconut oil in deep saucepan and sauté the celery and leek for 5 minutes until soft.
- Add the celeriac cubes and sauté for a couple of minutes longer.
- Add the water and bring the mixture to a boil then reduce the heat to simmer, covered, for 35 minutes, until the celeriac is tender.
- Blend the mixture until smooth either using an immersion blender or a food processor, working in

batches.

- Return the blended mixture to the pan and stir in the cream or coconut milk.

- Add more water if you prefer a thinner soup or continue to simmer if you prefer it thicker.

- Season to your liking with salt and pepper, then serve, garnished with parsley.

DINNER

Crockpot Mexican Pulled Pork

Prep time: 10 minutes

Cooking time: 10 hours

Servings: 8

Ingredients

4 lb bone in pork shoulder

2 Tbsp of smoked paprika

2 Tbsp of chili powder

2 Tbsp of ground cumin

1 Tbsp of ground black pepper

1 Tbsp of dried oregano

1 Tbsp of ground white pepper

2 tsp of cayenne pepper

1 full batch of Beasty BBQ Sauce

Instructions

- In a mixing bowl, combine paprika, chili powder, cumin, black pepper, oregano, white pepper and cayenne pepper. Mix it well. This will be your spice rub.

- Sprinkle the spice rub all over the meat and massage the meat gently, making sure to coat the meat with spice rub evenly.

- Wrap the meat in a plastic wrap for 3 hours or

overnight (you can refrigerate this for up to 3 days).

- When ready to cook, unwrap the meat and place in a Crockpot with ¼ cup of water.

- Cook on lowest setting for up at least 10 hours or until meat is fork-tender.

- Discard all the liquid in your Crockpot and transfer the meat in a cutting board.

- Shred the meat into thin shreds using two forks.

- Put the shredded meat back to the Crockpot and add in the BBQ sauce.

- Heat on lowest setting for 1 hour or until heated through.

Carrot & Cardamom Soup

Prep time: 10 minutes

Cooking time: 40 minutes

Servings: 6

Ingredients

1 Tbsp coconut oil or butter

2 large leeks, white and light green ends only, cleaned and sliced

Kosher salt

1½ lb carrots, peeled and cut into ½-inch rounds

1 apple, diced

1 tsp root ginger, peeled and minced

½ tsp ground cardamom

4 cups chicken stock or bone broth

½ cup coconut milk

Freshly ground black pepper

Instructions

- Melt the coconut oil or butter in a saucepan over a medium heat and add the sliced leeks and a couple of pinches of salt. Sautee for a 5 minutes or so until translucent

- Add the cardamom and ginger and stir for a minute or two until fragrant.

- Add the rest of the ingredients apart from the

coconut milk and bring to boil. Reduce the heat, cover the saucepan and simmer for 30 minutes.

- Blend the soup until smooth – either transfer to a food processor and process in batches or use an immersion blender.

- Season with salt and pepper and serve.

Citrus, Thyme and Rosemary Roasted Chicken

Prep time: 10 minutes

Cooking time: 1-2 minutes

Servings: 4-6

Ingredients

¼ cup of butter (melted)

1 whole chicken

1 onion, cut into large chunks

4-6 garlic cloves, smashed

1 orange or lemon, cut into 6 pieces

2-4 large carrots, cut into large chunks

1 tsp of kosher sea salt

1 tsp of dried thyme

1 tsp dried rosemary

black pepper to taste

Instructions

- Preheat oven to 350°F/180°C.

- Grease a bottom of a large roasting pan with half of the melted butter.

- Clean the chicken cavity, removing any gizzards or organs.

- Combine the onion, garlic and lemon in a bowl and fill the inside of chicken with the mixture.

- Place the chicken on a buttered roasting pan and arrange carrots around it.

- Brush the chicken with the remaining melted butter and season with the salt, herbs, and black pepper.

- Roast chicken until the thermometer inserted on the leg and breast reaches 165°F/75°C.

- Cooking time is approximately 20 minutes per pound, depending on the size of the bird.

Beef Rump Burgundy

Prep time: 15 minutes
Cooking time: 3 ½ hours
Servings: 6

Ingredients

¼ lb bacon, cut into short strips
4 Tbsp of butter
2 ½ - 3lb of beef rump roast, cut into 2-inch cubes
1 ½ tsp of salt
¼ tsp of pepper
2 Tbsp of almond flour
1 onion, sliced
1 Tbsp of tomato paste
2 cloves garlic, finely chopped
1 Tbsp of fresh thyme (or ¼ tsp dried)
1 Tbsp of fresh parsley, finely chopped
1 bay leaf
3 cups of full bodied wine such Cotes du Rhone or Chianti
2 ½ cups of beef stock
1 lb crimini mushrooms (white or brown), sliced

Instructions

- Preheat oven to 425°F/220°C.
- In a heavy saucepan, melt 1 Tbsp of butter and

sauté the bacon until cooked but not crispy.

- Add the beef to the bacon in 4 batches, until meat is brown.

- Transfer bacon and meat in a casserole baking dish.

- Season meat with salt and pepper and sprinkle with almond flour evenly.

- Bake uncovered for about 12 minutes, or until flour is absorbed into the meat forming a crust outside.

- Remove meat from the oven and lower the oven temperature to 325°F/165°C.

- Heat a heavy saucepan over the stove and melt 1 Tbsp of butter and add the remaining bacon fat from the bacon and meat and sauté carrots and onions until soft, about 7 minutes.

- Stir in the tomato paste, garlic, thyme, parsley and bay leaf.

- Pour in the wine and broth. Bring to a boil.

- Lower the flame and simmer for about 5 minutes, then pour this mixture over the meat in a casserole baking dish.

- Bake again in a hot oven, covered for 2 ½ hours. The cooking liquid should bubble gently while cooking.

- Check for doneness by pricking the meat with a fork, and it's done when meat is tender and can easily pulls meat apart.

- Meanwhile, heat the remaining butter in a saucepan

and sauté the sliced mushrooms.

- Don't crowd the mushrooms. Cook mushrooms in small batches, adding butter as needed, because according to Julia Child, if you cook too many mushrooms at once, it will be filled with liquid and won't brown. Set aside the mushrooms.

- Remove the casserole dish from the oven and pour the meat and its liquid into a colander, so the liquid drains out.

- Pour this liquid into a saucepan and simmer gently for 10 minutes. Pour over meat and mushrooms.

- Transfer meat into a platter and garnish chopped parsley and serve immediately.

Grain-Free Pizza

Prep time: 15 minutes
Cooking time: 25 minutes
Servings: 2 pizzas

Ingredients

Pizza Crust

1 ½ cups of tapioca starch or flour

½ cup milk

2 Tbsp of butter

½ tsp of salt

1 egg, beaten

¼ tsp of dried oregano

Pinch of white pepper

¾ cup of Parmesan cheese (or any hard cheese), grated

Pizza Topping

½ cup of pizza sauce

¾ cup of mozzarella (or other soft cheese)

Toppings

Instructions

- Add the milk, salt and butter to a saucepan and simmer over low heat until the mixture starts to bubble but not boil. Meanwhile, transfer the tapioca starch into a bowl.

- When the milk mixture starts to bubble, gently pour it into the tapioca starch and stir it all together - it will be clumpy, which is fine. If it seems too runny, keep adding tapioca starch until you reach the right consistency.

- Set aside the mixture to let cool, about 5 minutes, and preheat the oven to 500°F/260°C.

- When the mixture cools down, add the beaten egg and start kneading.

- Stir in the cheese and season with white ground pepper and oregano. Mix it all together until you form a soft dough.

- This dough is enough to make two pizzas.

- Divide the dough into two parts and stretch it out as thin as possible. Be careful to tear the dough, but pull it as far as you can.

- Place the dough in a cast iron skillet and use your fingers to spread it around the edges.

- Poke the dough with fork to create some holes to let the air pass through it.

- Place the skillet in the middle rack of your preheated oven and bake for about six minutes, then transfer the skillet over the stove top (but keep the oven on). At this point, the dough will have a bread-like appearance.

- Spread ¼ cup of pizza sauce over the crust surface.

- Add toppings of your choice, then put it back in the oven and bake for another 8-10 minutes or until the cheese starts to brown.

- Broil it for the last minute of cooking time if you want extra crispy toppings.

- You can also bake this pizza on a pizza stone or an ordinary baking sheet.

TREATS

Chocolate Chip and Cherry Cookies

Prep time: 15 minutes

Cooking time: 15 minutes

Servings: 15 brownies

Ingredients

1 cup almond butter

⅓ cup raw honey

1 egg, whisked

1 tsp vanilla extract

¼ tsp cinnamon

½ tsp baking soda

½ tsp baking powder

Pinch of salt

½ cup dark chocolate chips

½ cup cherries, sliced and pitted

Instructions

- Preheat oven to 350°F/175°C.

- Transfer all the ingredients apart from the chocolate chips and cherries to a mixing bowl and stir until the mixture is well combined. When well mixed, fold in the chocolate chips and cherries.

- Scoop the mixture in dollops onto a parchment lined baking tray using a cookie scoop or spoon – aim for 15 scoops.

- Bake for 15-17 minutes, allow to cool slightly and serve warm.

Blueberry Espresso Brownies

Prep time: 10 minutes
Cooking time: 30 minutes
Servings: 18 brownies

Ingredients

1 cup of Coconut Cream Concentrate (melted)
3 eggs
½ cup of Raw Organic Honey
1 cup of blueberries
1 cup of pecans, crushed
4 Tbsp of Organic Cocoa Powder
1 Tbsp of cinnamon
1 Tbsp of ground coffee (your choice)
2 tsp of vanilla extract
½ tsp of baking soda
¼ tsp of sea salt

Instructions

- Preheat oven to 325°F/165°C.

- Grease a 9x13-inch baking dish or mini-muffin pans with coconut oil.

- In a mixing bowl, combine coconut cream, eggs, honey, pecans, cocoa powder, cinnamon, ground coffee, vanilla extract, baking soda and salt.

- Mix all the ingredients until well blended, using a

hand/stand mixer.

- Gently fold in the blueberries, be careful so you don't crush the blueberries.

- Transfer mixture to your prepared baking dish or mini muffin pans and bake for 30 minutes.

- Five minutes before the end of baking time, test with a toothpick to judge the amount of baking time needed.

- Remove pan from the oven, let it cool then drizzle some coconut cream all over the brownies.

- Cut and serve. Enjoy!

Honey-Caramelized Figs with Yogurt

Prep time: 10 minutes
Cooking time: 10 minutes
Servings: 4

Ingredients

1 Tbsp of honey, plus more for drizzling
8 ounce of fresh figs, halved
2 cups of plain Greek yogurt
Pinch of ground cinnamon
¼ cup of pistachios, chopped

Instructions

- Pour honey in a non-stick skillet and heat over low-heat.
- Add figs, cut side down and cook until caramelizes, about 5 minutes.
- Serve caramelized figs over yogurt with a sprinkling of cinnamon and top with pistachios.
- Drizzle with honey before serving.

TWO THANK YOU GIFTS

As a Thank You to readers for buying this book we put together two free gifts to help you on your *Grain Belly, Wheat Brain* journey

These gifts were created for you to print off and keep handy in the kitchen, so visit the link below to get access.

www.BlueBeanpublishing.com/Gluten-Free

Heath Easton

DISCLAIMER/TERMS OF USE

Grain Belly, Wheat Brain
by Heath Easton

or indirectly.

The information provided in this book is for educational and entertainment purposes only. The author is not a physician and this is not to be taken as medical advice or a recommendation to stop taking medications. The information provided in this book is based on the author's experiences and interpretations of the past and current research available. You should consult your physician to insure the daily habits and principles in this book are appropriate for your individual circumstances. If you have any health issues or pre- existing conditions, please consult your doctor before implementing any of the information you have learned in this book. Results will vary from individual to individual. This book is for informational purposes only and the author does not accept any responsibilities for any liabilities or damages, real or perceived, resulting from the use of this information.

The information herein is offered for informational purposes solely, and is universal as so. The presentation of the information is without contract or any type of guarantee assurance.

The trademarks that are used are without any consent, and the publication of the trademark is without permission or backing by the trademark owner. All trademarks and brands within this book are for clarifying purposes only and are owned by the owners themselves, not affiliated with this document.

REFERENCES

[1] *F as in Fat*, Trust for America's Health and the Robert Wood Johnson Foundation, 2013 (www.healthyamericans.org/report/108/)

[2] *Prevalence of Overweight, Obesity, and Extreme Obesity Among Adults: United States, Trends*
[2] *Prevalence of Overweight, Obesity, and Extreme Obesity Among Adults: United States, Trends 1960–1962 Through 2007–2008*, Division of Health and Nutrition Surveys, 2010 (www.cdc.gov/nchs/data/hestat/obesity_adult_07_08/obesity_adult_07_08.pdf)

[3] *www.who.it* World Health Organization, 2014 (www.who.int/features/factfiles/diabetes/facts/en/index1.html)

[4] *International table of glycemic index and glycemic load values: 200,* Foster-Powell, Holt, and Brand-Miller, Am J Clin Nutr January 2002 vol. 76 no. 1 5-56 (http://ajcn.nutrition.org/content/76/1/5.full)

[5] *Scientists unlock the genetic secrets of bread*

wheat, Washington Post, 2014
(http://www.washingtonpost.com/national/health-science/scientists-unlock-the-genetic-secrets-of-bread-wheat/2014/07/17/8ee5768a-0dc9-11e4-8341-b8072b1e7348_story.html)

[6] *Identification of differentially expressed proteins between hybrid and parents in wheat (Triticum aestivum L.) seedling leaves,* Song X, Ni Z. Yao Y et al, Theor Appl Genet 2009 Jan;118(2):213-25. (www.ncbi.nlm.nih.gov/pubmed/18815767)

[7] *Malignancy and mortality in a population-based cohort of patients with coeliac disease or "gluten sensitivity* Anderson, McMillan et al, World J Gastroenterol. 2007 Jan 7;13(1):146-51. (http://www.ncbi.nlm.nih.gov/pubmed/17206762)

[8] *Increasing prevalence of celiac disease over time,* Lohi S, Mustalahti K, Kaukinen K et al. Aliment Pharmacol Ther 2007;26:1217-25

[9] *Non-celiac wheat sensitivity diagnosed by double-blind placebo-controlled challenge: exploring a new clinical entity,* Carroccio, Manseuto et al, Am J Gastroenterol. 2012 Dec;107(12):1898-90,

(http://www.ncbi.nlm.nih.gov/pubmed/228253 66)

[10] *Gliadin, zonulin and gut permeability: Effects on celiac and non-celiac intestinal mucosa and intestinal cell lines,* Drago, El Asmar et al, Scand J Gastroenterol. 2006 Apr;41(4):408-19. (http://www.ncbi.nlm.nih.gov/pubmed/166359 08)

[11] *Majority of Children With Type 1 Diabetes Produce and Deposit Anti-Tissue Transglutaminase Antibodies in the Small Intestine*, Maglio, Florian et al, Diabetes July 2009 vol. 58 no. 7 1578-1584 (http://diabetes.diabetesjournals.org/content/5 8/7/1578.long)

[12] *National Diabetes Statistics Report*, National Diabetes Education Program, 2012, (http://www.cdc.gov/diabetes/pubs/statsrepor t14/national-diabetes-report-web.pdf)

[13] *Autism Spectrum Disorder (ASD) Data and Statistics*, (http://www.cdc.gov/ncbddd/autism/data.html /)

[14] *A Gluten-free Diet as an Intervention for Autism and Associated Spectrum Disorders: Preliminary Findings,* P. Whiteley, et al., Autism 3, no. 1 (March 1999): 45–65, (http://aut.sagepub.com/content/3/1/45.abstract)

[15] *The ScanBrit randomised, controlled, single-blind study of a gluten- and casein-free dietary intervention for children with autism spectrum disorders*, Whiteley P, Haracopos D, Knivsberg AM et al, Nutr Neurosci. 2010 Apr;13(2):87-100 (www.ncbi.nlm.nih.gov/pubmed/20406576)

[16] *Depressed mood associated with gluten sensitivity--resolution of symptoms with a gluten-free diet,* Carr AC, N Z Med J. 2012 Nov 23;125(1366):81-2, (http://www.ncbi.nlm.nih.gov/pubmed/23254531)

[17] *Gluten ataxia in perspective: epidemiology, genetic susceptibility and clinical characteristics*, Hadjivassiliou, Grünewald et al., Brain. 2003 Mar;126(Pt 3):685-91. (http://www.ncbi.nlm.nih.gov/pubmed/12566288)

[18] *Randomised clinical trial: gluten may cause depression in subjects with non-coeliac gluten sensitivity - an exploratory clinical study.* Peters, Biesiekierski et al., Aliment Pharmacol Ther. 2014 May;39(10):1104-12. (http://www.ncbi.nlm.nih.gov/pubmed/2468945 6)

[19] *Opioid peptides derived from food proteins. The exorphins.* Zioudrou C, Streaty RA, Klee WA, J Biol Chem. 1979 Apr 10;254(7):2446-9. (www.ncbi.nlm.nih.gov/pubmed/372181)

[20] *High-fiber oat cereal compared with wheat cereal consumption favorably alters LDL-cholesterol subclass and particle numbers in middle-aged and older men*, Davy, Davy et al.,, Am J Clin Nutr August 2002 vol. 76 no. 2 351-358 (http://ajcn.nutrition.org/content/76/2/351.sh ort)

[21] *Atherogenic lipoprotein phenotype and diet-gene interactions.* Krauss RM. J Nutr 2001 Feb;131(2):340S-3S. (www.ncbi.nlm.nih.gov/pubmed/11160558)

[22] *A low-glycemic-load diet improves symptoms in acne vulgaris patients: a randomized controlled*

trial. Smith RN, Mann NJ, Braue A et al Am J Clin
Nutr 2007 Jul;86(1):107-15
(www.ncbi.nlm.nih.gov/pubmed/17616769)

[23] *Insulin-Like Growth Factor-1 Induces Lipid
Production in Human SEB-1 Sebocytes Via Sterol
Response Element-Binding Protein-1*, Smith, Cong
et al., Journal of Investigative
Dermatology (2006) 126, 1226–1232,
(www.nature.com/jid/journal/v126/n6/abs/57
00278a.html)

[24] *Clear Skin Diet, Chapter 3: Putting Out the
Flames of Can,* Alan Logan, Cumberland House
Publishing

[25] *The Dietary Intake of Wheat and other Cereal
Grains and Their Role in Inflammation*, Karin de
Punder and Leo Pruimboom, Nutrients. Mar
2013; 5(3): 771–787.
(http://www.ncbi.nlm.nih.gov/pmc/articles/PM
C3705319/)

[26] *Diet and Psoriasis: Experimental Data and
Clinical Evidence,* M. Wolters, The British Journal
of Dermatology. 2005;153(4):706-714.
(http://www.medscape.com/viewarticle/51410
8_4)

.

CPSIA information can be obtained
at www.ICGtesting.com
Printed in the USA
LVHW081010041019
633199LV00013B/212/P

9 781507 731130